Stretching Exercises For Beginners:

Increase Flexibility, Strengthen Your Body, Avoid Injury, Relieve Pain and Improve Overall Health

By

Charles Maldonado

Table of Contents

Introduction 5

Chapter 1. Initiating a Stretching Plan 6

Chapter 2. The Purpose of Stretching 7

Chapter 3. Types of Stretching 9

Chapter 4. Benefits of Stretching 15

Chapter 5. Stretching Tips 16

Chapter 6. Dangers of Stretching 19

Chapter 7. Common Stretching Exercises 21

Chapter 8. Stretching Tips for Older People 29

Conclusion 31

Thank You Page 32

Stretching Exercises For Beginners: Increase Flexibility, Strengthen Your Body, Avoid Injury, Relieve Pain and Improve Overall Health

By Charles Maldonado

© Copyright 2014 Charles Maldonado

Reproduction or translation of any part of this work beyond that permitted by section 107 or 108 of the 1976 United States Copyright Act without permission of the copyright owner is unlawful. Requests for permission or further information should be addressed to the author.

This publication is designed to provide accurate and authoritative information in regard to the subject matter covered. This work is sold with the understanding that the publisher is not engaged in rendering legal, accounting, or other professional services. If legal advice or other expert assistance is required, the services of a competent professional person should be sought.

First Published, 2014

Printed in the United States of America

Introduction

Stretching is an essential part of every workout plan. It reduces risk of injury, prevents sore muscles, and improves performance. When you stretch you are working the muscle fibers, which are attached to the stretch receptors of the muscle.

Beginning a stretching program will have great benefits in the long run. Your body will become healthier and you will be in better shape. Stretching exercises should be performed in an area where you have plenty of space and there won't be any interruptions, allowing for maximum potential.

Chapter 1. Initiating a Stretching Plan

Before starting to stretch one must warm up, a good way to warm up is by taking a 10 minute walk. When you begin a stretching routine ensure that you are stretching properly so as to avoid injury. Begin by doing the exercises a few times and as your muscles become more flexible you can increase your range of motion and length of time.

It is also important to pay close attention to your body. If a section of your body hurts while you are stretching, you should stop, at once. Stretches should only create slight strains, so it is very important you don't force yourself into a hard stretching exercise. Each stretching exercise should only take between 20 to 30 seconds. Movement should flow and a normal breathing rhythm should be maintained. Do not ever hold your breath while performing a stretch.

Include exercises that are not threatening to your body such as twisting your limbs in awkward positions. Additionally, to avoid having a monotonous workout schedule, add a wide array of routines.

Chapter 2. The Purpose of Stretching

When you stretch you lengthen your muscle tissues. This actions creates an increase in your range of motion, prevents injury and helps with rehabilitation. As part of your warm up and cool down process, stretching is essential.

Many people don't do their stretching before and after a workout plan. As a matter of fact, many skip stretching altogether because either time does not allow or there is a lack of motivation. This is unfortunate since stretching serves a purpose. The following are a number of reasons that stretching is purposeful.

1. Improving Flexibility – When you stretch, your muscles become more flexible and allow your joints to move in their complete range of motion (ROM). This full range of motion allows people to achieve the most out of their workout program. If you are going to engage in a vigorous stretching routine in order to improve flexibility, you should allow rest in between workouts.

2. Strength Training – Too much flexibility is bad for joints, but a moderate level stretching program will help deal with soreness during strength training. Waste removal is stimulated by lower intensity stretching.

3. Prevention of Injury – Repetitive movements can decrease range of motion. Stretching helps improve this problem, they should be incorporated into workout warm ups and cool downs.

4. Rehabilitation – Stretching can speed the healing process. It will be a slow and gradual process but it can help increase join performance. Be careful and don't overdo it. Overdoing stretching during rehab can cause more harm than good.

5. Technique – Keeping proper form, brings benefits. Static stretching calms the muscles and encourages stability.

Chapter 3. Types of Stretching

Though you may be familiar with stretching it is very important that you familiarize yourself with the proper techniques and terms. There is nothing wrong with learning more about the different types of stretches, since these terms are most often confused and misused. Stretching can be categorized in seven groups and they are: Static Stretching, Dynamic Stretching, Passive Stretching, Active Stretching, Ballistic Stretching, Isometric Stretching and PNF Stretching.

#1 – Static Stretching

This stretch is popularly used by runners. It simply means, that while stretching the individual maintains a section of the body and targets a muscle group while holding a position for a period of 10 to 30 seconds. Static Stretching is seen most in general fitness and is recommended as safe and very effective for increasing flexibility. Many professionals consider static stretching less productive than dynamic stretching for improving the range of motion (ROM) for physical activities such as sports and daily living.

An example of a static stretch is a toe touch. Sitting on the ground, legs stretched out forward, lift your arms straight over your head, bend at the waist and reach as far as you can and hold the stretch for 10 to 30 seconds.

#2 – Dynamic Stretching

Dynamic Stretching is achieved by going through a stimulating but pleasant stretching exercise with a repetition of 10 to 12 times. This type of stretching demands more careful coordination than static stretching because of the physical motions included. Physical therapists, trainers, coaches and athletes prefer this kind of stretching over static stretching since it reinforces the operational range of motion and mobilization in sporting activities and daily living. A dynamic stretching example would be:

- Leg & Arm Swings (Controlled)

- Torso Twists

Note well: Dynamic stretching should never be mistaken for the old-fashioned ballistic stretching, an example would be bouncing on your toes as given in PE Classes. Dynamic Stretching is manageable while ballistic stretching is uncontrolled, inconsistent, and bouncy. Although ballistic stretches have their advantages they should at all times be supervised since its risks override the benefits.

#3 – Passive Stretching

Passive stretching simply means that in order to achieve desired results during stretching you will be utilizing some sort of assistance. Your assistance could be in the form of your bodyweight, a resistance strap, gravity or another individual like a trainer. With passive stretching you loosen the muscles while waiting upon an external force to keep you in place. While stretching you most often may not have to work hard to do a passive stretch. Be aware that the external force may be stronger than your flexibility which can pose a risk and may cause injury.

An example of passive stretching is lifting your leg up and holding it on a ballet bar. The use of the bar to hold your leg during the stretch is the tool of assistance.

#4 – Active Stretching

Active stretching means that you are actively shrinking a muscle in contrast to the one you are stretching. With this type of stretching you don't use any other kind of external force as found in passive stretching. You are basically loosening the muscle because of the opposite muscle stretch. Active stretching can often times be challenging but is also regarded as low risk. With this stretch you are in control of the stretching force, it is determined by your own strength and flexibility.

An example of active stretching would be if you lift your leg high and hold it. Your leg will remain extended in this position without any assistance from another person or object.

#5 – Ballistic Stretching

This type of stretch uses the velocity of your moving body to push it past its accepted range of motion. Ballistic stretching is performed by bouncing in and out of a position, like a spring. This stretch is often associated with injury and is not widely used or accepted.

#6 – Isometric Stretching

Isometric stretches do not use motion like static stretches. This stretch tends to be more productive than both passive and active stretching alone. It is one of the best and fastest ways to increase flexibility. Strength is developed in the tensed muscles, because of resistance.

An example of Isometric Stretching is if you were to hold your foot and keep it from flexing, while at the same time your calf muscles are attempting to straighten your instep and point your toes.

#7 – PNF Stretching

This form of stretching is even more effective than isometric stretching at increasing flexibility. PNF stands for Proprioceptive Neuromuscular Facilitation. It is more of a method for joining passive and isometric stretching than a type of stretch. PNF was developed to help stoke victims rehabilitate. With this method the muscle will stretch passively and then contract against resistance isometrically while remaining in the stretched position. There are three common methods to this stretch:

- Hold-Relax

- Hold-Relax-Contract

- Hold-Relax-Swing

This type of stretching is more advanced and is not great for children. PNF Stretching should only be performed on a muscle group no more than once daily.

While there are seven types of stretching the most commonly used are a combination of these four types of stretches; active, static, dynamic and passive. Most of the stretches that are commonly seen and done are a combo of static and passive. Static and passive are the most popular stretches and the simplest to do. If done properly, these stretches will produce highly improved levels of flexibility and range of motion (ROM).

Chapter 4. Benefits of Stretching

Stretching can offer a number of benefits for those who choose to take the time to engage in the process. Some of these benefits are included below:

- Physical Performance will improve and your risk of injury will be lower.

- Body posture will improve.

- Increased Flexibility

- Lower back pains will diminish greatly.

- Better Circulation of blood and nutrients to your body tissues.

- Improved Range of Motion.

- Boost your total body coordination.

- Reduction in stress levels.

Chapter 5. Stretching Tips

Everyone wants to know how and when you should stretch. This next section will provide tips on when and how you should stretch.

Tip #1 - Stretch after your Workout Session: According to Research studies stretching before exercising will not minimize the risk of injuries and body aches. It is a known a fact that stretching out cold muscles could lead to pains in the body. If your aim is to heighten your flexibility, stretching your muscles after your workout is the best time since your muscles are warm. It is recommended to start stretching within five minutes of ending your workout, as it is the best time to enjoy stretching those muscles.

Tip #2 - Stretch the Muscles you targeted throughout your Exercising Session: If time doesn't allow for stretching at least stretch those muscles that you used during your workout. Focus on the muscles or group of muscles that may be the tightest, like the chest, calves, hamstrings, quads and hips.

Tip #3 – Stretch, Don't Bounce: When performing static stretches it best not to bounce. Remain in a position that is comfortable and stretch until you feel your muscles pulling gently. This should not hurt. Bouncing can result in pulled muscles or cramps.

Tip #4 - Perform Each Stretch for 15 to 30 Seconds: Stretching when your blood is pumping and your body is warm will majorly increase flexibility. A time frame of 15 to 30 seconds is ideal for a stretching exercise.

Tip #5 - Stretch during the Day: Stretch throughout your day. One of the benefits of stretching is stress reduction, stretching will deal with your stress during the day or even while you are at work.

How Often Should you Stretch to Improve Flexibility?

The question that is most frequently asked regarding stretching is, "How often and how long must one stretch in order to improve flexibility?" Many people guess that the more you stretch the better, but this is not completely correct.

Studies have shown that static stretching of each leg for 30 seconds a day, 3 times each week, for 4 weeks resulted in major increase of flexibility. This means that with just six minutes per month of stretching results were seen. Other studies discovered that 30 and 60 seconds of stretching had the same flexibility results. If you are a beginner it is recommended that you start at 30 seconds and work your way up to 60 seconds.

Chapter 6. Dangers of Stretching

Too much stretching or improper stretching are things to watch out for. Enthusiastic individuals who stretch improperly are not reaping all of the benefits. Some common mistakes while stretching are: incorrect warm-up exercises, insufficient rest between exercises, overstretching, doing the wrong exercises and in the wrong sequence.

It is of urgent importance to warm-up before stretching as the muscles are stretched best when they are warm. When done properly, warm-up exercises will loosen tight muscles and lead to an overall improved performance. In contrast, improper warm-up or none at all can greatly heighten the risk of injury when engaging in athletics.

You can also overstretch, when you stretch it's not just the muscles but the tissues surrounding the muscles that are stretched. These tissues are called fascial tissues. If they are stretched too much they lose their plasticity and as a result they are not properly functioning. Overstretching happens when you continue to stretch a muscle that has already been stretched.

Overstretching could result in:

-Torn Muscles

-Pain in the Tendons

-Back Pain

-Cramping

Below are a few common signs you could be overstretching:

1. Achy Muscles – A sign of overstretching could be constant muscle aches that are only made better by stretching.

2. Sciatic Pain – Daily pain in the sciatic nerve.

3. Clicking Joints – If your joints are always popping or cracking it is a sign of instability, possibly caused by overstretching.

4. Stiff Joints – Waking up with joints so stiff they cannot move properly. Often a sign that your ligaments have been overstretched.

Chapter 7. Common Stretching Exercises

- **Abdominal Stretch:** The main focus of this exercise is to stretch the abdominal muscles also known as the abs. When performing this workout you lie down face flat on the floor. Put your hands with palms facing down aligned with your shoulders. Straighten your arms and lift the top half of your body upwards and keep your head in line with your spine.

- **Supine Stretch Exercise:** This specific exercise aims on working out the muscles of your lower back. For this exercise, lie down flat on your back, with bent knees and feet against the floor. Then raise your knees upwards and embrace them towards yourself. Connect your hands behind your thighs and then pull your knees toward yourself. Hold them and after 30 seconds release them and repeat the same process.

- **Supine Hamstring:** When performing this stretching exercise you should lay down flat on your back with knees bent and feet on the floor. Hoist one leg into the air, keeping the leg straight but somewhat bent in the knee. Then place your hand around your leg while pulling it towards your chest and counting. After 30 seconds, you release and repeat the same drill.

- **Knee Extension:** Working out the shoulders is the core element to this exercise. While kneeling on the floor outstretch your arms in a forward motion. Stretch your bottom towards the heels but still keep the arms outstretched in front of you. Maintain this position for 15 seconds, release and redo.

- **Deltoid Stretch:** For this stretch lay flat on your back while bending your knees and feet on the floor. Keep your arm straight and bend it over your left shoulder, placing your right hand on the left elbow hoist your arm over. Keep that position and then let go. Then continue the same exercise with the opposite arm.

- **Lower Spine Stretching:** The goal of this exercise is to open the lower spine. Like the rest of the exercises you lay flat on the ground or floor. Lift your backside from the floor then roll your back down, as you do, move slowly and place each section of the back down.

Stretching Workout for the Office Environment

Sitting at a desk in an office all day long for five to six days a week and sometimes longer can be very detrimental to your body. If you have bad posture like; arching your shoulders or slouching in your chair can lead to pain. Common office related pain includes; headaches, backaches, neck pain, shoulder pain, and tightness of the body.

This section includes stretches that are ideal for the office environment. It targets groups of muscles and body parts like the neck, back, shoulders, hips and butt. Reduce some stress and ease some of that work related pain with these stretching exercises.

Chest Stretches: Since you spend a lot of time in the office hunched over. It is highly recommended that you perform chest stretches. To perform this exercise you will need a band. If you don't have a resistance band, they are easy to get at many sports stores. Easily store your resistance band at work for swift stretching and increasing strength. This exercise can be done either sitting or standing. Use the resistance band to create a wide stretch over your head, move your arms down and out as you stretch. Hold this stretch for 10 to 30 seconds. Do not try this stretch if you are exhibiting any kind of shoulder pain.

Shrugging Shoulders: Your neck and shoulders suffer stress, tension, and muscle knots from typing, and hunching over the desk. Office workers can benefit from this workout because shoulder shrugs help relax the shoulders and achieve a better circulation of blood flow. This exercise can be performed sitting or standing. Raise your shoulders to your ears, compressing them as solidly as you are able to. Keep the stretch for 1 to 2 seconds and bring them back down and relax. Continue for about 8 to 10 Reps.

Stretching your Upper Back: This section of the back becomes tight often and muscles need some dire exercising. Hunched shoulders can happen from holding the phone in between your head and shoulder and from the use of your computer mouse. To do this stretch you should be either seated or in a standing position, outstretch your arms and pivot your hands so your palms face out. While crossing the arms your palms must be squeezed together, engage the abdominals and back, reach away and relax your head. Maintain this stretch for 10 to 30 seconds.

Spinal Twist: Sitting inside your office for too many long hours can really affect your lower back, leaving it tight and aching. The Spinal twist will gently release that tension as you work out the lower back muscles. From a sitting down position place your feet flat on the floor or ground, engage the abs and gently turn your torso to the right side and use your hands as you hold on to the chair to intensify the workout. Only turn your body as far as you are able to, and keep your back straight and your hips intact. Hold for 10 to 30 seconds and repeat the stretch on the opposite side.

Stretching the Torso: Even those who are conscious of body posture are more than likely to slouch back unconsciously which can create back pains. This basic movement will warm up the group of muscles from your arms, sides and back. To do this stretch you need to be sitting down or standing with your hands together and fingers secured and pointing at the ceiling. Stretch high and inhale deeply, afterwards exhale and open your arms, bringing them back down. Repeat this activity for 8 to 10 Reps.

Stretching the Forearm: Do your arms every get tight from too much typing. The muscle group this stretch targets is the wrist and forearms. While sitting or standing, extend your arm as far out as you can and move your hand down with your fingers pointing down. Use your hand to tenderly pull the opposite hands fingers in your direction until you feel your forearm stretching. Hold your hand for 10 to 30 seconds, then repeat the process with the opposite hand.

Stretching your Neck: The neck is a highly affected area of the body. When tense, neck pains can result in serious back tension and headaches. Many office workers have the tendency to tilt their heads forward when sitting at a computer, this poses some added strain on the muscles. When performing these stretches positive effects will be felt on both the shoulders and neck. To do this stretch, sit down on a chair, then hold the chair with your hand and slightly pull while angling your head to the opposite direction. You will feel this stretch on the right side of the neck. Hold the pose for 10 to 30 seconds, redo the exercise on the opposite side.

Stretching your Hip flexor: The hips, and the lower section of your body is also affected from sitting down for long hours. When you sit the gluteus expands and the hip flexors get stiff. Outstretching this section of the body several times throughout the day can minimize the tightness one may feel. This stretch should be performed while standing up. Take your right leg and move it back as if you are about to spring out. Tighten you gluteus while bending the knees and lower yourself until you feel a stretch on the front area of your hip. Keep this position for 10 to 30 seconds and then do again on the opposite side.

Hip Stretches: This exercise works the complex group of muscles in the hips and butt. To perform this stretch you should be sitting down nice and tall, place your ankle on the opposite knee. Serenely, lean forward, maintain your back as straight as possible, reach out and stretch your torso until you feel the muscles in your right gluteus and hip stretching. To intensify this exercise add pressure to the right knee. Hold on for 10 to 30 seconds, alternate and repeat.

Stretching the Inner Thigh: Though this exercise may seem a little manly there is a positive relaxed effect on the groin, hips, and thighs. This is another hip activity that will also reduce tension, stress and strain on the muscles of the lower part of the body. To engage this stretch get into a sitting position, with your legs widened, and toes extended out. Then simply lean with elbows on your thighs. Keep your back straight and abdominals tightened. Tenderly press forward with the elbows and push on your thighs until you feel the stretch. Keep this position for 10 to 30 seconds, then repeat.

Chapter 8. Stretching Tips for Older People

After critical analysis and examinations, research studies, continue to proclaim that when it comes to exercising, age doesn't matter. In fact studies have revealed that elderly folks who stretch and exercise twice a week can strengthen their physical strength, flexibility, balance, coordination and agility significantly. Even minute improvements in physical well-being through activities can lengthen one's life and independent lifestyle.

A recent research found that men who extended their physical activities at 50 years of age, exhibited a reduction in rate of mortality that was the same as that of quitting smoking. As a matter of fact 10 years after having heightened their physical activities, these men had the same death rate for their age group of men who were physically active during their whole adult lives.

Here are some tips for older exercisers:

- See a Doctor. As an older person it is important to have a general physical and medical check-up, as well as professional guidance, before initiating any exercise program and even basic stretching exercises.

- Start low and slow. For older sedentary individuals one of the following programs may be recommended as safe and helpful to improving health. Low-transforming aerobics, gait training programs, Physical balance, Tai-chi, self-paced walking and lower leg resistance workouts. Nursing homes even provide workout plans that improve strength, equilibrium, gait, and flexibility that have remarkable advantages to enjoy.

- Try Stretching Exercises. Flexibility and stretching exercises for beginners helps foster healthy muscle growth as one is able to minimize the rigidity of the body and the loss of balance that comes with aging.

- Use a Chair. If you have trouble walking use a chair. Stretching exercises can be done with chairs.

Conclusion

Stretching is a necessary part of your workout routine. While it may seem insignificant it is not to be taken lightly. Stretches need to be done properly in order to ensure proper performance. Be sure to approach stretching with a warm up, so that your muscles can respond at their best.

If you find yourself aching the following day then there are signs that you either overstretched or did not follow instructions correctly. At the end of the day your main goal should be to achieve an increased level of flexibility that produces balance and a healthy body that will last for years to come. Overall if you apply the stretching routines the proper way you will be able to enjoy the benefits that stretching provides.

Thank You Page

I want to personally thank you for reading my book. I hope you found information in this book useful and I would be very grateful if you could leave your honest review about this book. I certainly want to thank you in advance for doing this.